Yoga
for
Digestion

12 Simple Yoga Exercises for
Enhancing Your Digestive Capabilities,
Improving Assimilation of Consumed
Food and
Shifting Your Metabolism into the Next
Gear

Advait

Contents

Disclaimer and FTC Notice

medical problems without the advice of a physician, either directly or indirectly.

The intent of the author is only to offer information of a general nature to help you in your quest for emotional, spiritual and physical well being. In the event you use any of the information in this book for yourself, which is your constitutional right, the author and the publisher assume no responsibility for your actions.

Under no circumstances will any legal responsibility or blame be held against the publisher for any reparation, damages, or monetary loss due to the information herein, either directly or indirectly. The information herein is offered for informational purposes solely, and is universal as so. The presentation of the information is without contract or any type of guarantee assurance.

Adherence to all applicable laws and regulations, including international, federal, state, and local governing professional licensing, business practices, advertising, and all other aspects of doing business in the US, Canada, or any other jurisdiction is the sole responsibility of the purchaser or reader.

Neither the author nor the publisher assumes any responsibility or liability whatsoever on the behalf of the purchaser or reader of these materials.

Any perceived slight of any individual or organization is purely unintentional.

The True Meaning of Yoga

There is a common and popular belief that 'Yoga' is an Indian ritual which is all about performing difficult physical exercises for maintaining health and curing diseases.

This is a MYTH!!

Actually, sound health is a side-effect of Yoga.

Surprising!!! But true.

The word 'Yoga' literally means *to unite ourselves with our higher self* - an entirely meta-physical objective which can be achieved through a Discipline of Physical exercises (Asana's) coupled with Meditation exercises (*Dhyana*) and Breathing exercises (Pranayam). When we perform those exercises we get in shape and achieve good health.

Yoga is not something which is only to be performed or practiced; it is also to be achieved.

Yoga is the destination and the path to it is through a disciplined practice of physical exercises, meditation and breathing exercises.

Maharshi Patanjali, in his revolutionary work *'Paatanjal YogaSutra'* prescribes an eight-fold path to achieve Yoga, known as *Ashtang Yoga*.

['Paatanjal YogaSutra' is considered to be the most comprehensive book on Yoga and it forms the basis and reference of all the Yoga methodologies practiced throughout the world today.]

The Ashtang Yoga [eight-fold path to yoga], given by Maharshi Patanjali is as follows:

Yama

The moral virtues that one should possess as they are considered to be essential for one's initiation on the path to yoga.

Niyama

It involves being knowledgeable and aware about your surroundings and then studying your-self to form an essential discipline which you would adhere to.

Asana

'Understanding and Performing' the required *physical exercises, this is the core of your yoga practice.*

Pranayam

It is all about breath control, which enhances the life energy which governs the existence of a being and balances the mental energy.

Pratyahar

Sensory inhibitions which internalize the consciousness and prepare your mind to take action.

Dharana

It involves inculcating an extended mental focus to concentrate on only those things that are essential.

Dhyana

It involves meditation, paying attention to your breathing and thus focusing only on yourself.

Samadhi

Becoming one with the object of your contemplation and experiencing spiritual liberation.

Yama and Niyama are essential for inculcating the needed discipline and to establish a strict routine.

Asana is the crucial physical part, which subjects your body to essential physical movements through different exercises.

Pranayam and Pratyahar are needed to guide us through the various breathing exercises and for making us aware of the internal spiritual changes as we ascend along the path to Yoga.

Dharana and Dhyana stages prepare us mentally and spiritually to concentrate inwards by using various meditation exercises.

Samadhi is the culmination stage where one achieves Yoga.

A Brief History of Yoga

Before going any further let's look back at where it all began.

To tell you the truth…. No one knows!!

The foundation of Yoga as a science is attributed to *Maharshi Patanjali* who lived in India in the 3rd Century B.C.

But, archeological excavations in the Indus Valley civilization sites have unearthed sculptures and idols depicting various Asana's (physical exercise positions) suggested in Yoga and these idols date back to around 3000 years B.C.

Also, information about various aspects of Yoga can be found in Vedic texts like; Shwetashwatrupanishad,

Chaandogyopanishad,

Kaushitki Upanishad,

Maitri Upanishad etc.

This information was scattered all over and Maharshi Patanjali, compiled these nuggets into a streamlined and strict science of Yoga or should I say he compiled this scattered information into a way of life called *Yoga* through his work 'Paatanjal YogaSutra'

After Maharshi Patanjali, Maharshi Swatwaram wrote 'Hatapradipika' (meaning - One Which Illuminates the Path of Hatha Yoga , i.e. the physical aspect of Yoga) in the 13th Century A.D.

And, Maharshi Gherand wrote 'Gherandsanhita' around the same time.

Almost all the Yoga methodologies practiced world-over today regard Maharshi Patanjali's work as their reference.

Importance of a Healthy Digestive System

If you are familiar with my previous works, you know that I like to keep all my books absolutely fluff free and concise. I promise you, this book will be no different.

I will not waste 15 pages in convincing you about how important it is for you to maintain a healthy digestive system. But, I will tell you what Ayurveda Says about the importance of proper digestion and assimilation.

Ayurveda states that, the health of an individual deteriorates as a result of breakdown of various essential organs due to fatigue, and in Ayurveda a fatigued stomach and digestive system are referred as the root cause of all ill health and disease.

In Ayurveda the process of digestion is broadly divided into 3 stages, viz.

#1 In the Stomach,

#2 In the Liver and

#3 In the Target Organs.

If the digestion in the Stomach is poor, the quality of digestion in the Liver is poorer and the digestion and assimilation in the Organs is the worst and this results in poor health and diseases.

Ayurveda states that *'Exercise removes the harm caused by most bad habits which most people have, and no movement of the body is as beneficial as body movements and exercise which aid in Digestion.'*

Exercise is the main principle in keeping one's health, and in keeping away all the illness.

The bottom-line is; a well established, sincere and disciplined Yoga practice aimed at improving your Digestive capabilities is Your body's first line of defense against any illness and disease.

Some Essential Precautions

Here are some precautions and rules you need to follow if you wish to achieve best results;

1. Yoga is very helpful if done in the Morning and on an empty stomach (don't eat anything, you can drink water). If you cannot make time in the morning, you can practice it in the evening but make sure that you practice it after 4 to 4 ½ Hrs. of having your meals.

2. When you get up in the morning , have a glass of water, visit the toilet, take a shower and then do Yoga, as water will rejuvenate your system and taking a shower will warm up your body for the exercises you are about to perform.

3. Understand this; You are the only essential for Yoga and not your clothes. I find all the recent 'yoga attire' fad to be pointless. All you need is a simple mat to sit on, A Pajama and a loose T-shirt which don't restrict your movements while you perform the Asana's.

4. Take your time while performing the Asana's, don't hurry through the exercises as if you are on a deadline. Remember, 'Yoga is for You...You are not for Yoga'. If you find yourself short on time, don't perform all the listed exercises in a hurry,

practice only a few that you can in that short time, but slowly and steadily.

5. Don't let your mind wander off while doing the Asana's, concentrate on your movements instead. A very easy trick is to concentrate on your breathing.

6. Women should not perform these asanas during menstruation.

7. A pregnant woman should not practice the Asana's from the 4th Month of her pregnancy.

8. Avoid performing Asana's back to back in quick succession, rest for at least 30 seconds between two Asana's.

9. After your Yoga session, do not eat or drink anything for at least 25 to 30 min.

10. If you have had a bone broken in the past and now it is mended, don't submit that appendage to too much strain while performing an Asana.

11. Commit to routine practice of Yoga, make it a way of life.

Yoga Asana #1

Vajrasan/Asana of the Thunder-Bolt

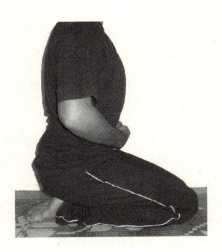

Method:

Stand straight with the waist, back and neck aligned and your feet around an inch apart.

Get down on your knees and fold your legs below your thighs.

Keep your feet spaced with the base of the feet (palms of the feet) facing upwards. (refer image)

(The nails of your fingers should touch the ground)

Then, place your bums on your heels.

While performing this Asana you can place your palms on your stomach as shown in the image or you can place them on your knees.

Duration:

This Asana (position) should be held for 25-30 seconds.

Repeat at least 3 times.

Other Benefits:

-This Asana enhances strength of your lower body.

-Regular practice of this Asana prevents the occurrence of kidney stones..

-It also strengthens the toes of your feet.

Yoga Asana #2

Manduk Asan/Asana of Frog

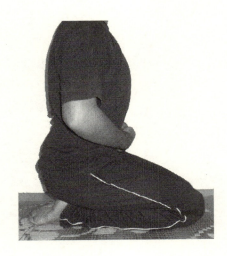

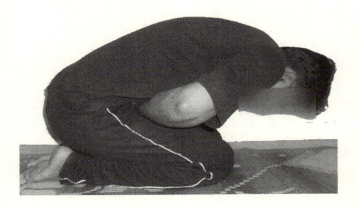

Method:

Sit in *Vajrasan* position.

Place your left palm on your belly button and then place the right palm over your left palm.

Exhale out completely and then suck in stomach as much as you can.

Then bend down your upper torso as much as you can. (you should be able to touch your nose to the ground with regular practice of this Asana)

Maintain this position for 8-10 seconds and then return to your previous Vajrasan position and then breathe in.

Duration:

This Asana takes 15-20 seconds to perform and you can repeat it 3 times.

Other Benefits:

-It keeps your pancreas healthy.

-It is very helpful in regulating levels of 'Insulin' in the body, thus is very helpful for people suffering from diabetes.

Yoga Asana #3

Ardh-Chandra Asan/ Asana of the Half-Moon

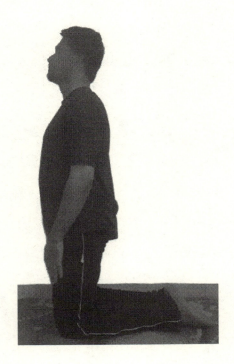

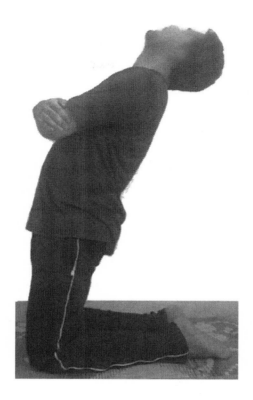

Method:

Sit in *Vajrasan* position.

Then lift your torso up and stand on your knees.

Fold your hands. (right hand over your left hand)

Then bend backwards as much as you comfortably can, while inhaling slowly.

Remain in this position for a few seconds and then come back to the original position while exhaling slowly.

Duration:

This Asana (position) should be held for few seconds.

Repeat at least 2-3 times.

Other Benefits:

- It is helpful in curing back pain.

-It is very helpful in relieving stress and anxiety.

Yoga Asana #4

Ardh Halasan/Asana of the Half-Plough

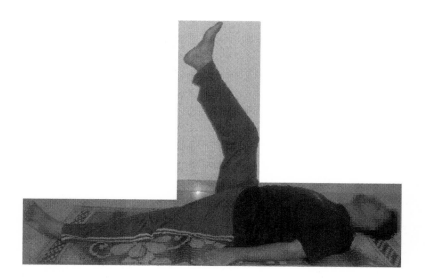

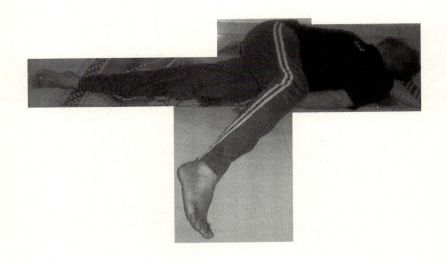

Method:

Lie on the mat/ground comfortably with your legs laid out straight and your palms should rest beside your thighs, palms facing down.

Slowly inhaling, raise your right leg straight up in the air. (Refer Image)

Hold your leg up for 3-4 seconds and then touch the ground to your left with your right leg, so that right thigh is resting on your left thigh, all the while maintaining your upper torso and hands in the original position. (Refer Image 2)

Maintain the position for a few seconds and then slowly exhaling, return to the original position.

(Repeat the procedure in the other direction, so that the left leg touches the ground and our left thigh is resting on your right thigh.)

This will complete one set of this Asana.

Duration:

Each set of this asana takes 10-12 seconds to perform and you can repeat it 3 times.

Other Benefits:

-This Asana reduces abdominal fat and is a very effective weight loss asana.

-It is very helpful in curing indigestion and gas problems.

-In women, this asana is very helpful in curing menstrual problems.

Yoga Asana #5

Ardh Matsyendra Asan/ Asana of Fish Lord II

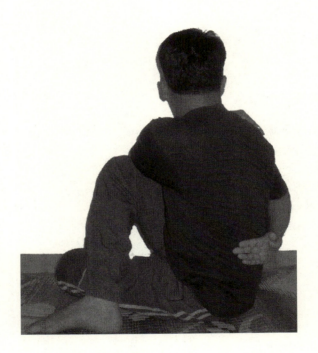

Method:

Sit comfortably on the mat with your legs stretched out front.

Fold your left leg under your right thigh.

Then, place your right leg on the outer side of your left thigh. (Refer Image)

Place your left palm on your right shoulder and place your right hand on your lower back in such a way that the back of your palm touches your lower back.

Slowly inhale, and then turn your upper torso to your right, as much as you comfortably can.

Remain in this position for 5-6 seconds and then come back to the original position while exhaling slowly.

Now repeat on the other side. [i.e. fold your right leg under your left thigh. Place the left foot on outer side of your right thigh. Place the right palm on your left shoulder and left hand should touch your lower back and then turn to your left.]

Duration:

This Asana (position) should be held for few seconds.

Repeat at least 2-3 times.

Uses:

-It is very helpful in strengthening your heart, lungs and liver.

-It is an excellent detox Asana.

Yoga Asana #6

Paad-Hast Asan/ Asana of Feet & Hands

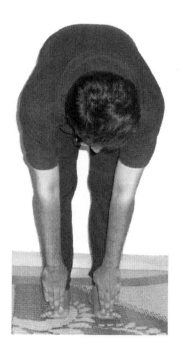

Method:

Stand straight on the mat with your feet together.

Now raise both your hands up, so that your fingers are pointing upwards and palms are facing forward.

Breathe in and then bend down and touch your toes with your respective hands.

(see to it that you are not bending your knees).

(You'll not be able to touch your toes at the start, but with regular practice you will achieve it)

Remain in this position for a few seconds all the while holding your breath in.

Then get to your standing position and exhale out.

Duration:

This Asana (position) should be held for few seconds.

Repeat at least 2 times when you start and then with practice increase the repetitions to 4-5 times.

Other Benefits:

-It works miraculously well in burning excess fat.

- It cures any stomach disorders you have.

Yoga Asana #7

Shashak Asan/Asana of Hare

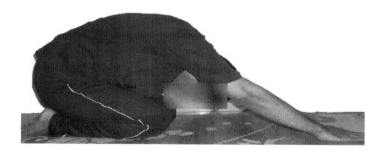

Method:

Sit in *Vajrasan* position. (refer the instructions of the 1st Asana)

Then raise both your hands up, so that your fingers are pointing upwards and palms are facing forward.

Your biceps should be touching your ears.

Exhale out completely and then suck in stomach as much as you can.

Then bend down your upper torso as much as you can. (your palms should be touching the ground/mat and also try to touch your forehead to the ground.)

Maintain this position for 3-4 seconds and then return to your previous Vajrasan position and then breathe in.

Duration:

This Asana takes 10-15 seconds to perform and you can repeat it 3 times.

Other Benefits:

-This Asana helps in toning the muscles of legs and thighs.

-It is very helpful in curing Arthritis and other neurological disorders.

Yoga Asana #8

Nauka Asan/Asana of the Boat

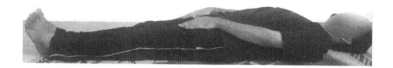

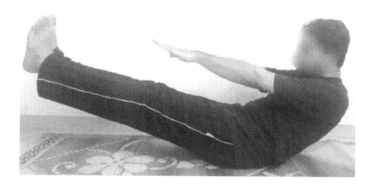

Method:

Lie on the mat/ground comfortably with both your hands resting on your thighs, palms facing down.

Then, slowly inhaling pull up your head and shoulders above the ground.

Then also raise both your feet, around 1 & a 1/2 foot in the air. (refer image)

(It is as if you are trying to touch your toes with your fingers)

Maintain this position for a few seconds, then slowly exhaling; come back to the original position.

Duration:

This Asana takes 10-15 seconds to perform and you can repeat it 3 times.

Uses:

-It strengthens your stomach and also helps in regulating blood sugar levels.

-It is very helpful for women as it helps cure menstrual problem.

-It also helps in strengthening your lungs.

Yoga Asana #9

Kati-Chakra Asan/Asana of Twisting Waist

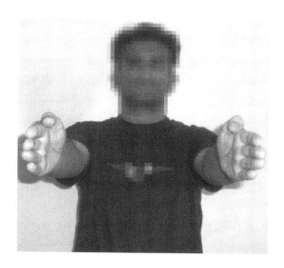

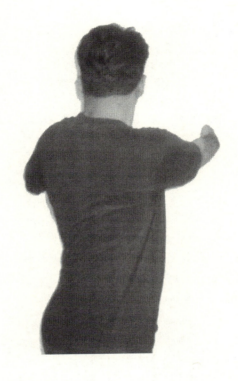

Method:

Stand straight on the mat with your feet, shoulder length apart.

Now, lift up your hands in front, so that they are parallel to the ground, and both the palms are facing each other. (Refer Image 1)

Then slowly inhaling, turn your upper torso to your left, as much as you comfortably can.

Look straight behind you. (Refer Image 2)

Hold this position for a few seconds and then return back to the initial standing position, while exhaling slowly.

Repeat the process, but this time turn your upper torso to your right.

This will complete one set of this Asana.

Duration:

Repeat at least 2-3 sets of this Asana.

Other Benefits:

-This Asana enhances the strength of your lower back.

-It is also very useful in curing any neck disorders.

-Regular practice of this Asana improves the function of your thyroid gland.

Yoga Asana #10

Tadasan/Asana of Palm Tree

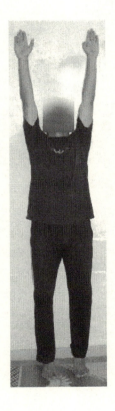

Method:

Stand straight on the mat with your feet together.

Now raise both your hands up, so that your fingers are pointing upwards and palms are facing forward.

Take a deep breath and don't exhale. (*Kumbhak*)

Now raise your heels up from the ground by putting all your weight on your toes. (refer image)

Hold this position for 3-4 seconds, then return to the normal position and exhale out slowly.

Duration:

This Asana takes 10-12 seconds to perform and you can repeat it 3 times.

Other Benefits:

-It is very effective in strengthening your spine.

-It strengthens your limbs.

-It is a very effective Asana for curing constipation.

Yoga Asana #11

Dhanurasan/Asana of the Bow

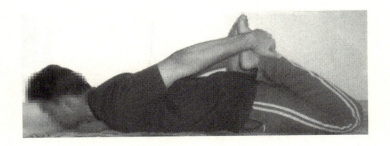

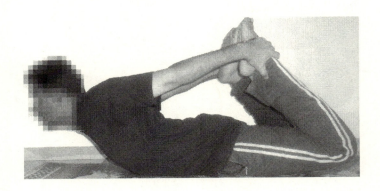

Method:

Lie down on the mat/ground facing down, i.e. your stomach, chest and chin touching the ground, with your hands at your side, palms facing down.

Now fold your legs, so that your heels touch your bums.

Then hold your ankles with your respective hands. (Refer Image)

Take a deep breath, hold it in.

Lift your shoulders and chest above the ground with the help of your legs.

Hold this position for a 4-5 seconds and then slowly exhaling return to the initial position.

Duration:

This Asana takes 8-10 seconds to perform and you can repeat it 2 times.

Other Benefits:

-It strengthens your back.

-It also helps in maintaining the health of reproductive organs.

-It also increases the functionality of your lungs and thus helps in curing respiratory disorders like Asthma.

Yoga Asana #12

Shalabh Asan/Asana of Locust

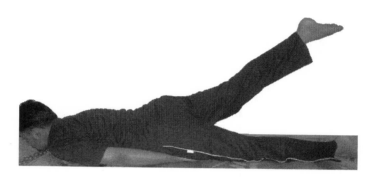

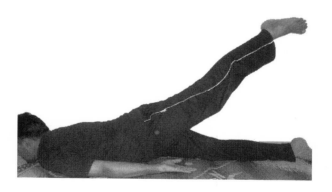

Method:

This Asana is to be done lying down.

Lie on your stomach with your chin placed on the ground/mat.

Your feet should be close together and the nails of your toes should be touching the ground.

Slide your palms under your thighs.

Raise the right leg in the air, hold it up for 3-4 seconds and bring it back down.

Then raise the left leg in the air, hold it up for 3-4 seconds and bring it back down.

Duration:

This Asana takes 12-15 seconds to perform and you can repeat it 3-4 times.

Other Benefits:

-It makes the spine, waist, back muscles and blood vessels flexible.

-It is also helpful in increasing your concentration.

Thank You!

Thank you so much for reading my book. I hope you really liked it.

As you probably know, many people look at the reviews on Amazon before they decide to purchase a book.

If you liked the book, please take a minute to leave a review with your feedback.

60 seconds is all I'm asking for, and it would mean a lot to me.

Thank You so much.

All the best,

Advait

My Other Books
On Mudras

Mudras for Awakening Chakras: 19 Simple Hand Gestures for Awakening & Balancing Your Chakras

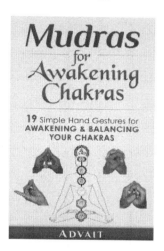

http://www.amazon.com/dp/B00P82COAY

[#1 Bestseller in 'Yoga']

[#1 Bestseller in 'Chakras']

Mudras for Weight Loss: 21 Simple Hand
Gestures for Effortless Weight Loss

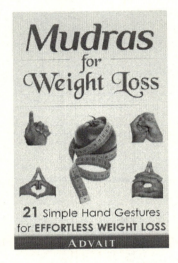

http://www.amazon.com/dp/B00P3ZPSEK

Mudras for Spiritual Healing: 21 Simple Hand Gestures for Ultimate Spiritual Healing & Awakening

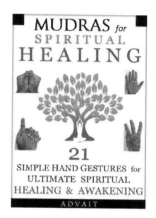

http://www.amazon.com/dp/B00PFYZLQO

Mudras for Sex: 25 Simple Hand Gestures for
Extreme Erotic Pleasure & Sexual Vitality

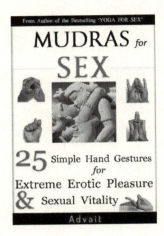

http://www.amazon.com/dp/B00OJR1DRY

Mudras: 25 Ultimate techniques for Self Healing

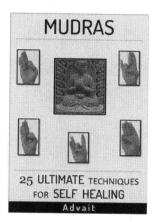

http://www.amazon.com/dp/B00MMPB5CI

Mudras for a Strong Heart: 21 Simple Hand
Gestures for Preventing, Curing & Reversing
Heart Disease

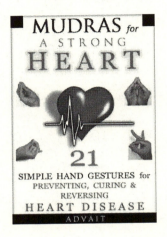

http://www.amazon.com/dp/B00PFRLGTM

Mudras for Anxiety: 25 Simple Hand Gestures for Curing Your Anxiety

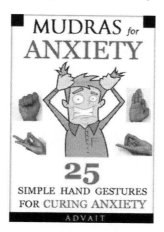

http://www.amazon.com/dp/B00PF011IU

Mudras for Memory Improvement: 25 Simple Hand Gestures for Ultimate Memory Improvement

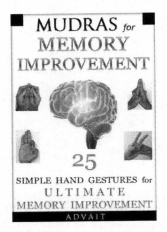

http://www.amazon.com/dp/B00PFSP8TK

Mudras for Stress Management: 21 Simple Hand
Gestures for a Stress Free Life

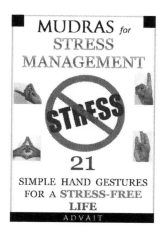

http://amazon.com/dp/B00PFTJ6OC

Mudras for Curing Cancer: 21 Simple Hand
Gestures for Preventing & Curing Cancer

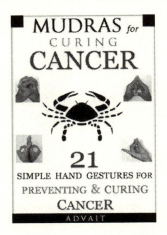

http://www.amazon.com/dp/B00PFO199M

On Yoga

Easy Yoga: Your Ultimate Beginners Guide to Understanding Yoga and Leading a Disease-Free Life through Routine Yoga Practice

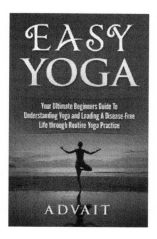

http://www.amazon.com/dp/B010I97366

Monday Yoga: Pranayam and Sukshma-Asana's for starting Your Routine Yoga Practice and Inducing Vigor into Your Life on the first day of the Week

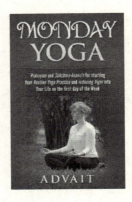

http://www.amazon.com/dp/B011SI6MK4

(This book is available for FREE)

Tuesday Yoga: 12 Yoga Asanas to be performed on Tuesday as a Part of Your Daily Yoga Routine

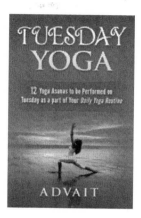

http://www.amazon.com/dp/B013GGA1AS

Wednesday Yoga: 12 Yoga Asanas to be performed on Wednesday as a Part of Your Daily Yoga Routine

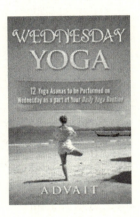

http://www.amazon.com/dp/B014RTDQ5U

Thursday Yoga: 12 Yoga Asanas to be performed on Thursday as a Part of Your Daily Yoga Routine

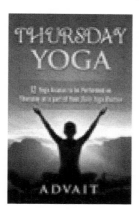

http://www.amazon.com/dp/B015JMSEPQ

Friday Yoga: 12 Yoga Asanas to be performed on Friday as a Part of Your Daily Yoga Routine

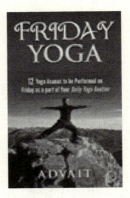

http://www.amazon.com/dp/B015UK17KG

Saturday Yoga: 12 Yoga Asanas to be Performed on Saturday as a Part of Your Daily Yoga Routine

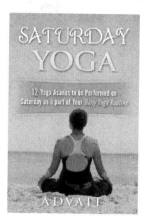

http://www.amazon.com/dp/B0165WFUJW

Sunday Yoga: Suryanamaskar (Sun Salutation) & 5 Yoga Asanas for a Blissful Culmination of Your Daily Yoga Routine

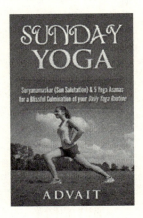

http://www.amazon.com/dp/B016Q8GF8K

Made in the USA
Middletown, DE
07 May 2017